HOW VACCINES WRECK HUMAN IMMUNITY

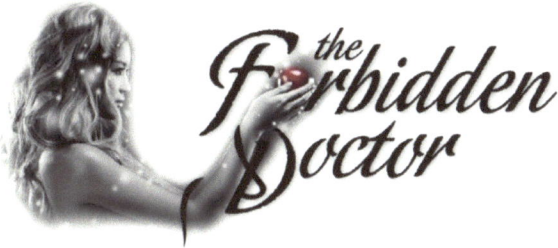

A Forbidden Doctor Publication

www.ForbiddenDoctor.com

E. Jackson Stockwell, DC CGP
NUCCA Board Certified
Certified GAPS Practitioner

Mary H. Stockwell, CGP ACN
Certified GAPS Practitioner
Applied Clinical Nutritionist

Copyright

Other books by Dr. Jack and Mary Stockwell:

Melting Breast Lumps (http://amzn.to/1J53uVV)

WARNING AND DISCLAIMER

The statements in this book have NOT been evaluated by the FDA (U.S. Food & Drug Administration).

Information provided here and products sold on ForbiddenDoctor.com and/or JackStockwell.com are not intended to diagnose, treat, cure, mitigate or prevent any specific disease or offer an assessment of a specific health condition.

The information provided by these sites and/or by this eBook is not a substitute for a face-to-face consultation with your physician, and should not be construed as medical advice of any sort. It is a list of resources for further self-research and work with your physician or health-care professional. Anyone who wishes to embark on any dietary, drug, exercise or other lifestyle change intended to prevent or treat a specific disease or condition should consult with and seek clearance from a qualified health-care professional.

Contents

HOW VACCINES WRECK HUMAN IMMUNITY

Nobody likes to think they have been brainwashed. But when you get through reading this eBook some of you are going to be very angry, and you're going to know you've been "had." This is the vision of the Forbidden Doctor,™ to let you know that there are alternatives to the medical status quo. The reason we use the term "forbidden" is because the powers that be in modern "Health Care" go to great lengths to keep this knowledge from you. These great lengths include character assassination, threats and follow through of licensure removal, denial of bonus' and/or pensions and retirement, or even imprisonment and death. There have been many prominent researchers, who when they made discoveries contrary to the party line, have just disappeared.

Thank goodness for current whistle blowers inside the CDC, the NIH, independent medical research, and the major 501C3 tax free charitable societies which comprise a list too long to put into this eBook and other so called organizations dedicated to your so called health. When in fact, many of these just continue the same old party line that health can only be obtained from a bottle or a knife.

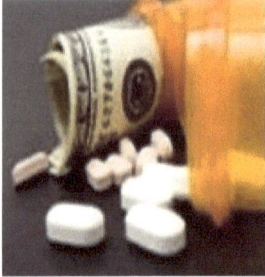

We don't have "healers" in our country anymore; we haven't for over a century, we just have a business, called "Health Care."

We have been raised in our culture to accept the voice of authority as the final word, even when they're wrong. Anything less would be heresy. This attacks our very value to discover we may be wrong about our foundational understanding of health and healing, but even more so, our deepest sense of value is stripped from us when we realize we have in fact, been brainwashed. Not through any fault of ours, however, we were raised to believe and trust the voice of authority. Is there a greater authority than a white coat with a stethoscope hanging around it?

We all think we would never fall for brainwashing. Consider this analogy: You have a little five year old child, whom you have convinced there are monsters in Canada, maybe because you were told there were monsters in Canada. If you told them this often enough, even when they had evidence to the contrary, by the time they reached adulthood they would still suspect this was true. It would take a lot of explaining, unlearning, teaching and fact finding to get them to understand otherwise. And still, they might be very apprehensive to take a vacation to that beautiful land. It might take years to dispel the lies that they were told so often. And even then, they may never visit Canada...they may find self-validating reasons to stay where they are, and never venture to that "scary" land. This would be a safe non-confrontational way for them to never learn the truth. And yet, the brainwashing would still have had its effect.

The purpose of this eBook is to help you to understand that the suppression of symptoms is not true healing in any sense of the word; which bring us to the concept of vaccinations. This provides the perfect forum for understanding the difference between words like "curing, healing and prevention" according to their definition, and true curing, healing and prevention, that only the body itself can perform. Interestingly enough, the courts have decided the medical world is the only one that is legally allowed to use these terms. This devolves these incredible words into legal terms and not terms related to health.

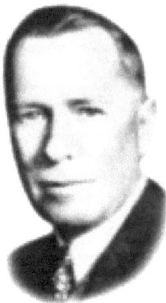

"One of the biggest tragedies of human civilization is the precedence of chemical therapy over nutrition. It's the substitution of artificial therapy over natural, of poisons over food, in which we are feeding people poisons trying to correct the reactions of starvation."
- Dr. Royal Lee, 1935

The point we're trying to make, is it's not that you don't have enough Prozac in your blood stream that is causing the symptoms of depression. The underlying concept here is that we first turn to a chemical based answer for immediate results, rather than discovering the underlying cause of depression. Which gets the cart before the horse.

Even still, many run to drugs to "solve" their symptoms of depression. Actually very, very few dare go against the years of training in their youth and venture out into that unknown hinterland of true healing. But that is what The Forbidden Doctor is all about.

REVEALING THE LIES YOU HAVE BEEN TOLD YOUR WHOLE LIFE

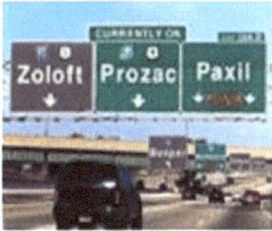

"It's not you don't have enough Prozac in your blood stream that is causing the symptoms of depression." - Dr. Jack

Let me give you an example: Dr. Royal Lee, the founder of Standard Process, the whole food supplement company we use in our clinic, tried to sell the product Zypan™ in 1937 - as a digestive aid. The FDA forbade it, even though Zypan is composed of the best digestive enzymes available. Camel Cigarettes, in 1937 (the same year) was allowed to sell their cigarettes - as a digestive aid. Can you believe that? That is because our health care system is just a business. The pharmaceutical companies knew that if you started smoking cigarettes they would have a patient in 20 years or so - it was a long term investment. But if you healed your digestion, they knew they would have less patients for all the reasons we go to a doctor.

So they bought out the senators and congressmen with campaign contributions to their re-election campaigns, paid the lobbyists, and passed a law that effects all people outside of Big Pharma and the medical profession that says in essence, If we, in our clinic, mention a disease connected with a nutritional protocol

11

or nutrient, we can go to jail for 20 years! If we ever said an apple can help a particular disease - we're a goner. That's a federal law and is "on the books" in every state. So what I'm going to tell you about vaccinations and immunity is a very closely held secret. A secret so powerful they have put out disseminating lies - such as mercury is put into shots as a preservative, so that their business they call "health care" can make billions. All this, at the expense of you and your children.

Question: How do you defeat a bad idea?

Answer: With a better idea.

You have been sold and sold and sold, and sold over again, that there is something wrong with your body. And that a happy, healthy decent life is not possible without the addition of chemical substances.

So we are going to lay out some simple facts, some education, some basic concepts about your magnificent immune system, things you have never been told.

The most fun thing in the world is learning something new, something that shakes your world.

You have been kept in the dark and systematically lied to, and have been propagandized through collusion between Big Pharma and the federal government concerning your body's ability to heal, repair and live in beautiful harmony with viral and bacterial entities along with the rest of the unseen microbial world.

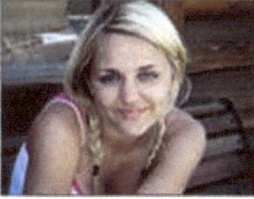

".... your body is set to repair and restore, not degenerate."

We're going to try to make this very simple, yet exciting at the same time. Most of what you are about to read comes from *Guyton's Physiology*, 10th edition, the unimpeachable source of how our bodies work...which is pretty dry reading, but it is where an understanding of our immune system begins. So here comes the new information - the forbidden information kept from you. So to get away from the fear, and have a sensible discussion, you must realize this, your body is SET to repair and restore, not degenerate. And it works in beautiful cooperation with all of nature if left alone to do so. All you need to do is water and feed it and give it plenty of rest. If you will do these things, employing clean water and wholesome organic food, it will take quite good care of you, as it has done for thousands of generations.

Perhaps the most important regulatory processes in the human body, are those that help you to live in harmony with the macro and micro world. This system of processes is known as the "Immune System."

IMMUNE SYSTEM

To understand how vaccines wreck the immune system, we need to get down to business.

Did you know if somebody comes within 2 feet of you, your skin turns a little acidic, to ward off any bacteria?

Our bodies have three types of immunity:

1. Infant Immunity
2. Innate Immunity
3. Acquired Immunity, or Humoral immunity

First of all there is **infant immunity**, the one you were born with. About the middle of the second trimester of your development, which would be around 20 weeks, some of your mother's antibodies passed across the placental barrier into your blood stream. As far as modern science knows, in your mother's womb, your developing body is completely sterile. Your blood is clean and so is your gut, free from any bacterium or virus. You will not encounter them, for the most part, until you are born. So in the second half of your fetal development these antibodies, which you received from your mother, are floating in your blood stream and will be ready to act when you take your first breath.

You received these from your mother because your body will not have the ability to make these antibodies until you are around 12 months of age - this is important to know. After six months, the mother's antibodies you were born with begin to decrease as your own infant immunity begins to strengthen. This is why you rarely hear of infectious diseases like diphtheria, measles, and polio ever bothering an infant in the first sixth months of their life, unless this beautiful orchestra is somehow disrupted by outside influences such as antibiotics and/or other medicines, heavy metals, environmental toxins, and especially vaccines at any time during the first year of life. The thing to remember here is babies don't have the ability to create antibodies until around the 12th month. So why are we injecting virus' into their little bodies?

Any honest immunologist, communicable disease specialist, or public health official will tell you why babies are vaccinated prior to one year of age. It is simply to train the parents to bring their children into the doctor's office for inoculations.

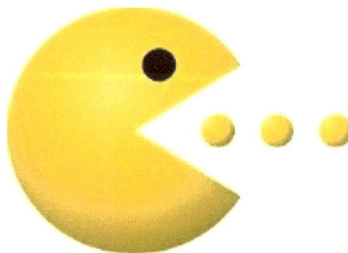

Next, there is your **"innate" immunity**. It is called innate because it was there from the beginning of your life and it is running all the time in the background, 24/7. The primary members of this system are the phagocytes, the PacMan of the lymph and blood stream, constantly on patrol throughout the fluids of your body looking for "not self", those "things" that do not belong there.

Another part of this immunity is the very hot acid in the stomach that kills off most of the microbial lifeforms that come into us through our diets. Your stomach acid should be as hot as battery acid, on constant guard, like the moat around a castle, drowning and destroying any life form that would love to get past that barrier.

Then you have what is called the acid mantle of the skin. Your outer covering should have a pH of 4.5 to 5.5. This "lake of fire and brimstone" that covers you is not felt by you at all, but is death to the billions of life forms falling on you every day.

Finally there is a soup of other chemicals and compounds in your blood stream, and in and out of your cells called lysozymes, polypeptides, compliment complex, NK cells (Natural Killer cells), etc., constantly on guard fighting the enemy and defending your life all the time, awake or asleep.

Now the "biggie", the fun one, the one that is always in the news, the one we believe lies at the heart of all the autoimmune disease explosion, the most perfect part of the inner intelligence inside you that the vaccine industry has laid waste to, is known as **acquired**

immunity or humoral immunity, the learning and adapting part of your immune system. This is the one the medical industry, either does not trust or does not believe will work on its own, and needs drugs to be effective. This is the crowning blessing that Mother Nature gave you to defend yourself against disease, and at the same time, the one the medical industry cannot leave well enough alone. 'If it ain't broke, don't fix it." Well, they broke it. They broke its back...with the chemical inoculations we call vaccinations.

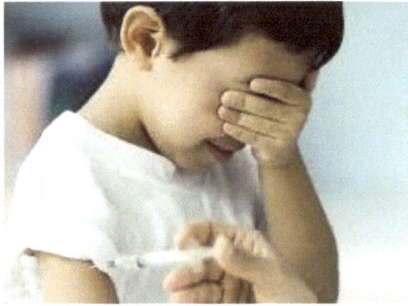

This acquired immunity is the part I want you to understand. This knowledge will give you the ability to talk to your family, your doctor and the nurse at the county health department where you will go get your exemption form for vaccinations, to protect your baby's beautiful immune system.

There are two types of acquired immunity and they are easy to understand and explain:

1. Cell mediated immunity that we will be referring to as **T Cells**

2. Humoral immunity that we will be referring to as **B Cells**

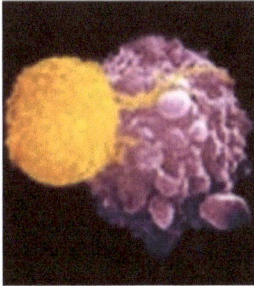

T cells, search out,

attack and destroy

There is more to acquired immunity than just T cells and B cells, but for the sake of this eBook we will leave it at that.

To understand the effect of vaccinations on the immune system, you have to understand the difference between these two forms...T Cells and B Cells.

T Cells - These cells recognize a virus or bacteria, as an antigen, and attacks and destroys them on contact. In a healthy immune system they act without hesitation and their destroying force is swift, effective and final. This is what makes up pus in an infection, both the dead invader and the T Cells. T Cells are called T cells because even though they are born elsewhere in the body they are schooled and trained in the thymus gland. They are very effective killers. They have no morals, they have no political beliefs, they have no religious agenda...they see something that doesn't belong and they neutralize and kill it, such as a chicken pox virus, or a pneumonia causing bacteria, or any of thousands of invaders, most of which you've never heard of. You get the idea.

So that's T Cells, they search out, attack and destroy. We mention T Cells first because they are the first to act. B Cells, or humoral immunity, do not do their thing until after the devastation left by the T Cells. It can take the T Cells seven to 14 days to destroy the enemy. Which is why it usually takes two weeks to completely get over a cold.

B Cells - are to T Cells what the CIA is to our Armed Forces. The B Cells are in the background watching and observing what the T Cells have done. B Cells are not activated until the T Cells start doing their work - this is important. B Cells do not attack or destroy the enemy. These are the cells that produce antibodies based on chemical messengers from the T Cells (and other cells we are not addressing here) which give the B Cells the codes to produce antibodies. What this means is, should that invader ever appear again, the antibodies are present to alert the whole immune system, even quicker this time to destroy the enemy before it gets a foot hold. It can take 14 to 28 days for B Cells to manufacture antibodies once they are called into action. Once these antibodies are formed you have life-time immunity to whatever triggered that T Cell reaction and will not get "sick" again from this antigen.

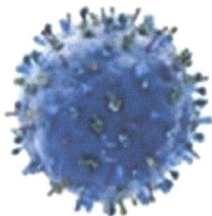

B cells produce antibodies based on chemical messengers from the T Cells

Let's talk about being what we call "sick"

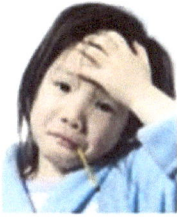

It's not the viral bacteria entity that makes you sick. It's your body's reaction to their presence that makes you sick.

If we have such great immune systems why do we get sick in the first place? This may come as a shock, but it's not the viral or bacterial entity that makes you sick. It is your body's reaction to their presence that makes you sick. Your body will beg, borrow and steal everything it can to keep your blood, your lymph and your cells clean and healthy. So when you are exposed to a virus or bacterium your body releases a whole cascade of chemical messengers to get rid of this antigen.

It begins with an attack by the T Cells. Mast cells release histamine to begin the inflammation process, (thus inflammation is usually good).

Digestive processes are altered to expel the enemy through vomiting, diarrhea, mucus excretions, or excessive sweating. Chemical messengers will trigger the liver to increase body temperature to destroy the invader - we call this a fever. Prostaglandins mount a chemical attack against the enemy, this can cause systemic pain - we call this headache, sore throat, stomach ache, muscle ache, intestinal ache, etc. It is not the enemy making you sick, it is your body making you "sick" to get rid of the enemy. This may be the first time you've ever heard this!

We always think it is the bugs, the germs, which make us sick. But in reality, it is our own body that make us sick. Dr. BJ Palmer, over a hundred years ago, said: "If the germ theory of disease was true, there would be nobody left alive to believe it." This is not to say there are not dangerous germs out there, it means that if the disease process was simply the matter of being exposed to germs, and since we are all exposed to germs all the time, we would all have died by now.

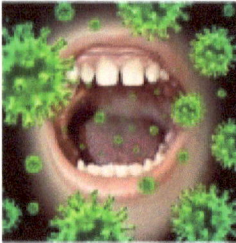

"If the germ theory of disease was true, there would be nobody left alive to believe it."
- Dr. B J Palmer

We understand there are very serious sicknesses, and many, many deaths, caused by your body's ineffectiveness to fight off the invaders. We understand how deadly this is and the subject is not to be taken lightly. Just the discussion of vaccinations has caused divorce and such horrible anger and fear that is almost unapproachable - after all it is the life of your children we are talking about. So we don't take this discussion lightly.

There have been now, as of this date, January 2015, over 10,000 deaths from Ebola alone. But many people have lived through the infection. This topic is so forbidden there are laws against even discussing it without rock solid, FDA approved disclaimers. But this extreme seriousness is the very reason it <u>must</u> be discussed. We must find the answers. We must. We must find the best answers to prevent death from microbes, and to strengthen our immune systems. And maybe most importantly, we must not cause harm to anyone in the process. This is the very reason for this eBook. We must be brave.

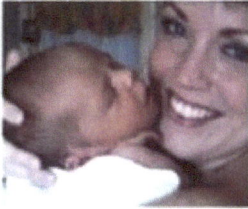

We must find the answers. We must. We must find the best answers to prevent death from virus', and to strengthen our immune systems.

A good review of patients that have succumbed to deadly virus' will show a weakness in their nutritional status and a plethora of medically prescribed drug use - be that vaccinations or medicines.

So every naturally occurring sickness has both T Cell and B Cell reactions. Such as chicken pox. The virus gets in your body, you have a cell mediated response (T cells). You get sick, blistery, feverish, then the humoral response (B Cells) begins and you never get chicken pox again, even when exposed multiple times. You never know it even happened again. Both of these aspects occur, in that order, always.

Remember...as nature designed. First the T Cell reaction, then the B Cell reaction.

THE CALCULATED DISRUPTION OF YOUR IMMUNE SYSTEM

> The whole point of vaccines is to stimulate the humoral response- B cells, without the cell mediated- T cells response first. This is the quintessential getting the "cart before the horse."
>
> -Dr. Jack

Prior to 1940 this beautifully orchestrated system of self-defense against the outside world worked wonderfully well for thousands of years. There are of course exceptions when a pandemic spread through the land. These were caused more by political influences than these disease process itself, but that's a subject for another book. However, it is because of this beautifully orchestrated system that we continue to live on this planet in the presence of an inconceivable number of the "enemy," almost entirely unseen.

Something has been happening since 1940. Since WWII we have seen a virtual explosion of autoimmune diseases, neurodegenerative diseases, stunning digestive dysfunction, cardio pulmonary disease, and the worst of all, cancer. Autism has virtually gone pandemic as two decades ago the autism rate was one in 10,000. In some areas of our country it is one in 22. At the current rate, we predict by 2020 it will be one in two.

We believe a major causative factor is vaccines. The whole point of vaccines is to stimulate the humoral response - B Cells, without the cell mediated - T cell response first. This is the quintessential getting the "cart before the horse."

This has to be understood to understand vaccines. They skip the natural process of cell mediation, where you get "sick", and go straight to antibody formation.

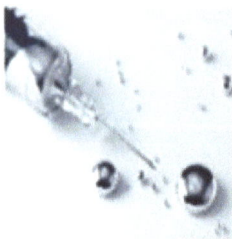

...one would wonder why you would ever inject mercury into a living human being? You have been told it is a preservative. This is like calling cyanide a preservative!

Think about it...if vaccines stimulated the cell mediated response first, the kids would get sick when you vaccinated them. What parent is going to take their kids to a doctor that makes them sick? So they had to figure out a way to stimulate humoral mediation without making you sick. They couldn't put a live virus in you, or you would get sick and nobody wants to be injected with a live virus anyway.

So they figured out a way to use a dead, or a weakened (attenuated) virus, and bypass T Cell mediation, and go straight to B Cell antibody formation. Now on the surface this appears to make a lot of sense. This is like having your cake and eating it too. You can't have both. In other words, can you change the natural order of things, genetically determined for thousands of generations, and come away without some serious side effects? Remember the commercial, "You can't fool Mother Nature"? We are of the opinion that this is the very thing Big Pharma is trying to do, fool Mother Nature. We are afraid we have become the "fooled."

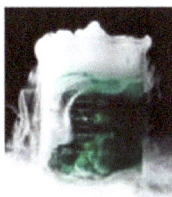

"So when they tell you they have taken out the mercury, they have only upped the content of the aluminum."

How can a vaccine jump the first step and go to the second with no ill effects on our genetic makeup? Well it can't. And it hasn't. And we are in for a tsunami type awakening during the next generation or sooner.

So since a vaccine only has a dead virus involved, which would not trigger a T Cell reaction, it was necessary to shock the system with chemical additives, called adjuvants, to force the body to mount a B Cell, humoral, antibody formation. These adjuvants, also known as excipients, are: mercury, aluminum, formaldehyde, etc.

27

Mercury, being the most naturally occurring neurotoxic substance known to man, one would wonder why you would ever inject mercury into a living human being. You have been told it is a preservative. This is like calling cyanide a preservative! Deadly poisons do not preserve, but they do have another function in smaller dosages. They literally shock the nervous system into reacting to the dead, or almost dead virus by producing antibodies.

So when they tell you they have taken out the mercury, they have only upped the content of aluminum and/or formaldehyde, and or polysorbate 40, etc., all of which are neurotoxic! So you are no safer. The vaccines are NOT "green." That's why vaccine makers laugh when people demand safer vaccines. That is the very purpose of the mercury or other adjuvants, to create a neural shock to the immune system! Without this chemical force the immune system would not recognize the dead or attenuated virus. So that is quite different than referring to mercury as a preservative.

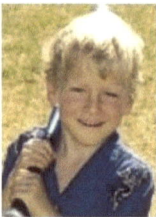

How did something virtually unknown- autoimmune diseases- before 1940 become the #1 debilitating process today?

This obviously is not how the body was designed to operate, however, there is no other way around it! Since we have been on this planet the immune system couldn't care less about a dead virus, so the violent neurotoxic chemicals were put into the vaccine cocktail to force the body to recognize it. Can there be an action without a reaction? No. "Every action has an opposite and equal reaction" according to Sir Isaac Newton.

So what might the opposite reaction be to shocking the immune system with an adjuvant such as, aluminum, mercury, formaldehyde, etc.? How about antibodies? How about lots and lots and lots and lots and lots of antibodies, from lots and lots and lots and lots of vaccines? **Just what are those antibodies going to do with no virus to attack?** Thus the autoimmune disease explosion, where all these unnaturally formed antibodies attack you.

So since the 1940's, if you do this enough, to enough people, to enough kids, over and over, you will get a suppressed T Cell mediated response and a heightened B Cell humoral response. The whole order gets upside down. Why?? Because that was the intention! The very goal! To bypass the "sick" part, and give us an unnatural immunity to virus'.

So what happens is this: Cell mediated immunity - T Cells, go on vacation. And the humoral immunity - B Cells, go through the ceiling!

Make a list of diseases that we are seeing all the time now without a T Cell mediated response (the "sick" part of disease)...they just happen spontaneously...asthma, allergies, eczema, Crohn's, colitis, MS, Parkinson's, Sjogren's, Hashimoto's, and more. These diseases are all marked by increased autoantibody production without cell mediation. This is what an autoimmune disease is.

All these diseases come on suddenly in some cases, in others, over a while, with slow onset of symptoms <u>but there never is any sickness that proceeds it</u>. The diseases we are always hearing about in the news now did not start with fever, vomiting, diarrhea, headaches, body aches and rashes. These diseases were diagnosed by the presence of autoantibodies in the blood stream. An autoantibody is where you have an antibody attacking you, yourself - not some microbe!

This was absolutely unheard of prior to WWII! And now even the Debakey Institute in Houston, Texas, the developers of the heart bypass operation, says that ALL heart disease is all autoimmune. This is also the largest area of current medical research, with over 80 identified autoimmune diseases in the human body. How did something virtually unknown - autoimmune diseases - before 1940 become the #1 debilitating disease process today?

An estimated

24 MILLION AMERICANS

suffer from one or more of over

80 AUTOIMMUNE DISEASES

This is staggering information.

Remember when most of us were children, there were almost no children who were sick? At what point did you first hear about Autism? Probably in the last decade. How about all these children with brain tumors, diabetes I and II, juvenile arthritis, including rheumatoid arthritis and cancers in almost every organ in their body? Almost out of nowhere we now have 20-40% of our children chronically sick and ill. Do you know not one person died of asthma before the 1950's? Well, I was born in 1950 and I don't remember anybody ever being sick except one kid that had asthma. That's it! One kid. We played in the dirt, in stagnant ponds, in mud, we didn't wash our hands before eating. Well, sometimes, and we didn't get sick. Oh, we had an occasional cold, or stomach flu, or chicken pox, that triggered the beautiful cell mediated response of the T Cells, but I didn't know anybody that died or was chronically sick. Their body saw the enemy, attacked the enemy and set up an antibody defense that will last to the end of their lives.

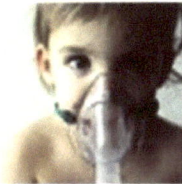

Do you know not one person died of asthma before the 1950's?

Since measles is hot in the news right now, here's a little tidbit of some more forbidden information from 1959: From the British Medical Journal, (www.bmj.com) the oldest medical journal on the planet:

> *"In the majority of children the whole episode has been well and truly over in a week, from the*

prodromal phase to the disappearance of the rash, and many mothers have remarked "how much good the attack has done their children," as they seem so much better after the measles". In this practice measles is considered as a relatively mild and inevitable childhood ailment that is best encountered any time from 3 to 7 years of age. Over the past 10 years there have been few serious complications at any age, and all children have made complete recoveries. As a result of this reasoning no special attempts have been made at prevention even in young infants in whom the disease has not been found to be especially serious. (Vital Statistics, British Medical Journal, February 7 1959, p. 381)

Below, is a link to a CNN video clip where cancer was cured by injecting a woman with the measles virus. Key in the browser URL link below to view the video on YouTube:

https://www.youtube.com/watch?v=DTLL6IMf8NY&feature=youtu.be

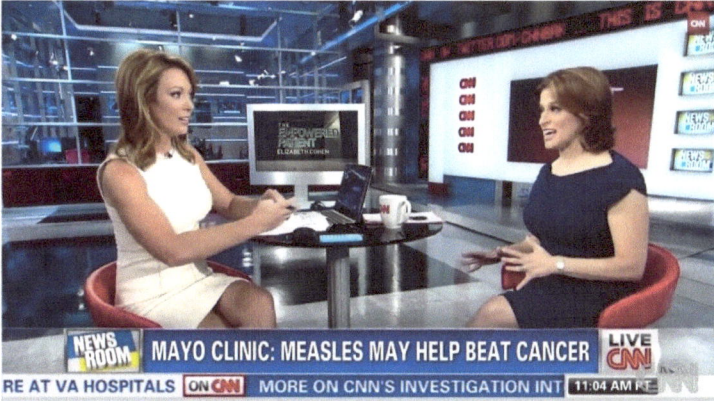

If you listen closely in the video you will hear them say that injecting the patient with the measles virus didn't have the same effect as a natural exposure to the virus! You need to understand this. Natural acquired immunity, not chemically forced immunity, is the best way to immunize yourself.

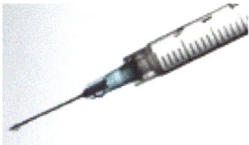

Injecting the patient with the measles virus didn't have the same effect as when naturally acquiring the virus.

A study in Kobe, Japan, showed that mice could develop an autoimmune disease by using several repeated vaccinations. Some say, "Well, that hasn't happened in humans," but it has over the last 70 years of vaccinations!

THEN THERE'S THE BIG POLIO HYSTERIA…

Almost every website you go to on this topic and more books than we can mention in this report, point to the fact that the overwhelming majority of diseases of which we have a vaccine were almost eradicated before the vaccine showed up. As shown in the graphs below.

Prior to the appearance of the Salk and Sabin vaccines for polio, the disease was almost 90% eliminated from the public scene.

"No epidemics of polio have occurred in the United States since 1954. The Salk vaccine was introduced in 1955, Sabin's in 1959. There is no evidence that the vaccines caused polio to practically disappear from this country." Vaccination, Examining The Record, page 56 - Judith A. DeKava

Graphical evidence shows vaccines didn't save us:

Polio

Diphtheria

Scarlet Fever

Whooping Cough

Measles

Typhoid Fever

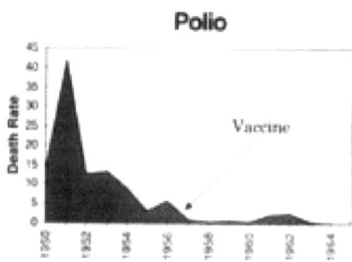

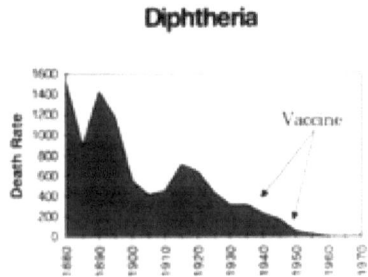

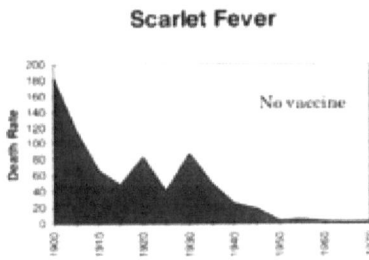

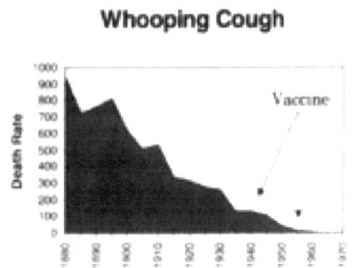

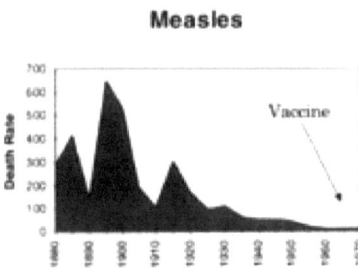

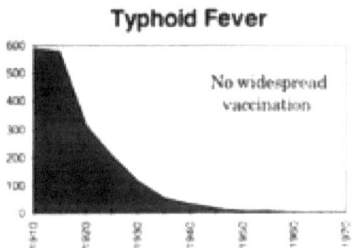

The above graphs, are based on the official death numbers as recorded in the Official Year Books of the Commonwealth of Australia, and represent the decline in death rates from infectious disease. They clearly show that vaccines had nothing to do with the decline in death rates.

The same statistics happened in the United States:

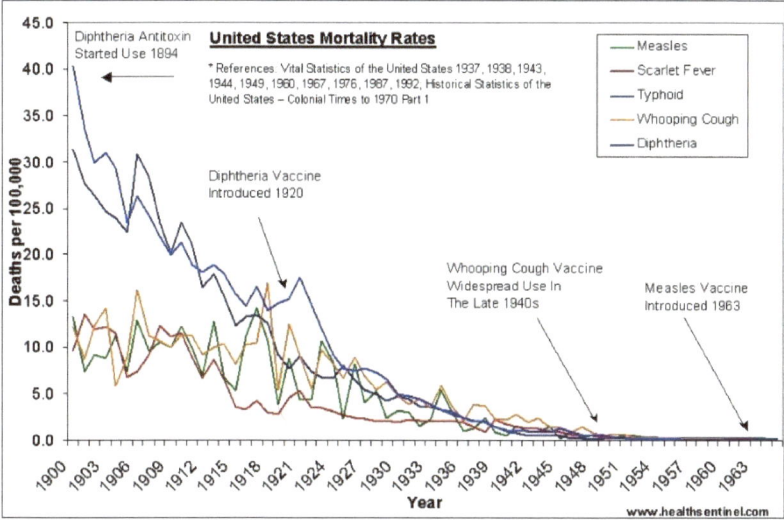

United States Mortality Rates

* References: Vital Statistics of the United States 1937, 1938, 1943, 1944, 1949, 1960, 1967, 1976, 1987, 1992, Historical Statistics of the United States – Colonial Times to 1970 Part 1

Diphtheria Antitoxin Started Use 1894

Diphtheria Vaccine Introduced 1920

Whooping Cough Vaccine Widespread Use In The Late 1940s

Measles Vaccine Introduced 1963

Legend: Measles, Scarlet Fever, Typhoid, Whooping Cough, Diphtheria

www.healthsentinel.com

So what were the true reasons for this decline? From his book 'Health and Healing' Dr. Andrew Weil best answers it with this statement:

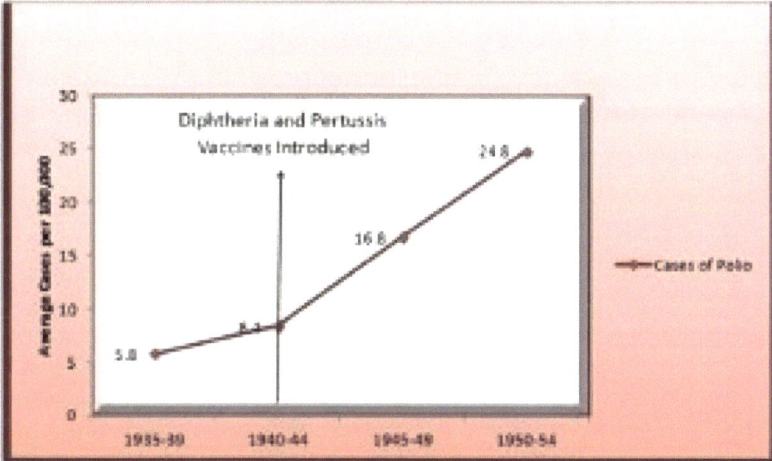

Diphtheria and Pertussis Vaccines Introduced

Cases of Polio

When diphtheria and pertussis vaccines were introduced in the 1940s, cases of paralytic poliomyelitis skyrocketed¶

37

"Scientific medicine has taken credit it does not deserve for some advances in health. Most people believe that victory over the infectious diseases of the last century came with the invention of immunizations. In fact, cholera, typhoid, tetanus, polio, diphtheria and whooping cough, etc., were in decline before vaccines for them became available - the result of better methods of sanitation, sewage disposal, and distribution of food and water."

The thing you have to understand, is the main culprit of polio was high sugar intake by its victims. In the early 1950's South Carolina called for a voluntary significant reduction of sugar consumption by the citizens of the state. Whereupon, the State of South Carolina immediately experienced a 90% reduction of polio.

In fact, Dr. Salk himself said, *"When you inoculate children with the polio vaccine, you don't sleep well for two or three weeks."* At that point, one would wonder with the already significant decrease in the incidence of polio throughout the country by this time, why one would inoculate a child anyway?

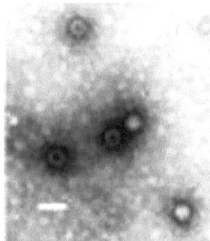

Polio Virus

And how did we deal with Polio before the 1940's? Here's how: *"The Polio virus enters the body by nose or mouth, then travels to the intestines where it incubates. Next, it enters the bloodstream where "anti-polio" antibodies are produced. In most cases, this stops the progression of the virus and the individual gains permanent immunity against the disease."* (Okonek BM, et al. Development of polio vaccines. Access Excellence Classic Collection, February 16, 2001:1. www.accessexcellence.org/AE/AEC /CC/polio.html)

Ah hah! So that wonderful, nature ordained, T cell and B cell natural immunity works again!

ISSUES TO CONSIDER

So there are basically 3 issues to consider:

1. **Do vaccinations work?** If a naturally acquired immunity creates a lifetime immunity, why do we need boosters after being inoculated? As shown in the graphic below, there is not any evidence or controlled trials proving they do any good at all. Take a look at the actual insert taken from a Flu vaccine (www.VaxTruth.com).

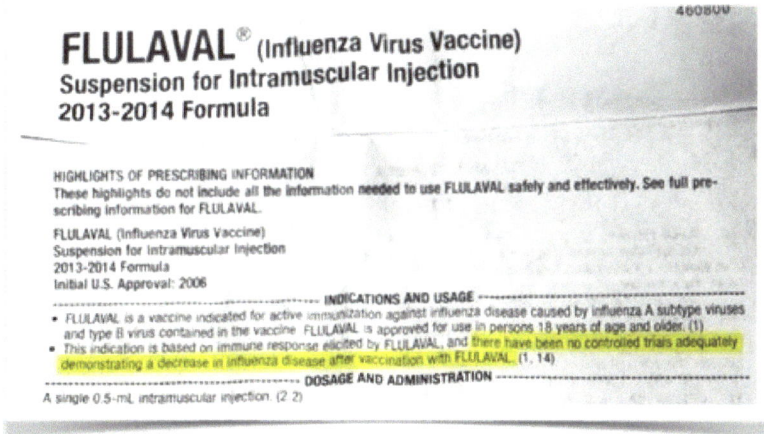

460800

FLULAVAL® (Influenza Virus Vaccine)
Suspension for Intramuscular Injection
2013-2014 Formula

HIGHLIGHTS OF PRESCRIBING INFORMATION
These highlights do not include all the information needed to use FLULAVAL safely and effectively. See full prescribing information for FLULAVAL.

FLULAVAL (Influenza Virus Vaccine)
Suspension for Intramuscular Injection
2013-2014 Formula
Initial U.S. Approval: 2006

---------------- INDICATIONS AND USAGE ----------------
- FLULAVAL is a vaccine indicated for active immunization against influenza disease caused by influenza A subtype viruses and type B virus contained in the vaccine. FLULAVAL is approved for use in persons 18 years of age and older. (1)
- This indication is based on immune response elicited by FLULAVAL, and there have been no controlled trials adequately demonstrating a decrease in influenza disease after vaccination with FLULAVAL. (1, 14)
---------------- DOSAGE AND ADMINISTRATION ----------------
A single 0.5-mL intramuscular injection. (2.2)

2. **What about injecting neurotoxins through all the barriers of the human body directly into the blood stream?** Can this be good? Is there a fair trade off in this that you would inject a neurotoxic substance that will get through the blood brain barrier and

41

into the brain itself in exchange for not getting the chicken pox? Or measles? Or mumps? Really?

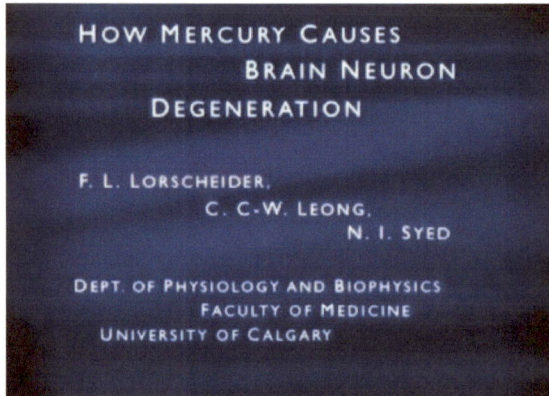

HOW MERCURY CAUSES
BRAIN NEURON
DEGENERATION

F. L. LORSCHEIDER,
C. C.-W. LEONG,
N. I. SYED

DEPT. OF PHYSIOLOGY AND BIOPHYSICS
FACULTY OF MEDICINE
UNIVERSITY OF CALGARY

Type in this URL in your web browser to view the video on YouTube:

https://www.youtube.com/watch?x-yt-ts=1422503916&v=XU8nSn5Ezd8&x-yt-cl=85027636

3. Where are all these autoimmune diseases coming from? What has happened in the natural order of things that the immune response would be turned upside down, in that your body is now attacking itself rather than the microbe?

Dr. Jack Stockwell debates Dr. Paul Offit on Vaccines

No too long ago I was invited to debate Dr. Paul Offit on national radio concerning the effectiveness of juvenile vaccinations. This happened before an audience of 4 million people. As the expert in alternative medicine on the National Doug Stephan Good Day Radio Talk Show Program (www.dougstephan.com), I invited Dr. Offit to speak first. Dr. Offit, the Chief of Pediatric Diseases at Baltimore Children's Hospital, is known nationally as "Dr. Vaccination." He is the poster child of the CDC's recommended program of over 150 inoculations between birth and age 18.

He began his speech in the usual way, haranguing the audience about the complete and total safety of multiple inoculations during any one doctor visit. He said the risks were minimal, of little consideration when compared to the great benefit provided by the vaccination that children would not get sick anymore.

(At this point, from reading this eBook this far, you know that the "getting sick part" - cell mediated immunity, is vital to the overall process of natural immunization, and cannot be skipped without consequences.)

Following a short commercial break it was my turn.

I only had one thing to say, and it went like this, "Dr. Offit, you know there are no long term studies that prove vaccinations are safe and effective one way or the other. From the 1940's until now nowhere in this country or any other country on the globe, are there any established long-term studies showing that a vaccinated child is healthier than an unvaccinated child, or vice versa." Where upon he immediately interrupted me and said, "That is not true, there are long term studies."

At this point I said, "Dr. Offit would you be so kind as to provide me with those long term studies?" I have to admit I was shocked to hear this because after many years of study on this subject I have never found long term studies. I should say that by long term, medical research considers that to be 10 years or more.

Much to my surprise Dr. Offit answered my request and forwarded to me a "long term" study. It was one he performed himself on 15 children at his hospital over a period of 14 days. In this study these children were injected with a vaccine and demonstrated the presence of antibodies to that injection within 14 days.

This hardly constitutes a long term study, in fact it was insulting to my question on national radio. No wonder he didn't quote this on the air.

I chose out of respect for Dr. Offit, to not embarrass him by telling the audience he is the owner of many vaccine patents and has made millions of dollars from these patents. To this day, there are still, no long term studies, essential to an established scientific protocol, involving vaccine efficacy, as the insert shown above for the flu vaccine Flulaval indicates.

So it comes down to this...

What is the potential benefit of injecting a child or adult with a known neurotoxin with immune shifting chemicals? There is not an issue as to if it will happen, it does happen; this shifting toward autoimmunity. It does not always rise to the level of a life destroying disease, but you cannot repeatedly vaccinate someone and expect their immune system to react properly.

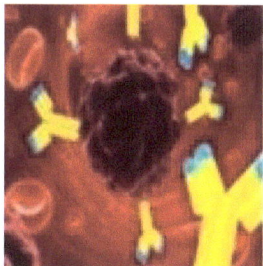

There is not an issue as to if it will happen, it does happen; this shifting toward autoimmunity.

So knowing this you have to decide what you are going to do. To quote Thomas Cowan, M.D. (http://fourfoldhealing.com), *"I think it is a rational decision for a parent to say, I know that giving my child a chicken pox vaccine will turn their immune system backwards, it will shift them toward allergies, autoimmune diseases, and even cancer. I know it will create some neurotoxicity...but I am just not willing to face the chance of them getting chicken pox. Fine."*

We have talked to patients in our clinic who say that very thing... Dr. Thomas Cowan continues, *"What I don't like is the health department, the hospitals, pediatricians saying vaccines work great and there is no downside. Hogwash. I mean that's a fairy tale. So long as parents and adults know both sides of the story, they can make their own decision."*

So, are all microbes bad for you? Is it necessarily a bad thing when some sickness overcomes us and we are bed ridden for a few days? Do we have to mount a constant attack of disinfecting every surface in our houses every time we turn around? Do we need to turn back anyone we meet anywhere from touching us we might suspect to be sick? To be honest, I would rather have a two week flu than to be injected with a mercury laden cocktail right into my blood stream. Don't be deceived - flu vaccines contain mercury.

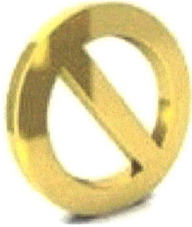

Here is the Forbidden GOLD: There are no good or bad viruses.

Now here is the Forbidden GOLD: There are no good or bad viruses. We do not live on an island. We live among them. They live among us. We are meant to live in a community of living things, the large and the very small.

Just think about it, as a child grows, they don't want to cuddle, they push away from us to get down on the floor. They are very serious about this, and they put everything in their mouths so as to become "one" with the viruses and microbes. They know instinctually if they don't, they will die. This is how they self-immunize, driven by the marvelous innate intelligence within their bodies. Young new mothers have been brainwashed into sterilizing the binky's, bottles and blankets to their child's detriment believing that the slightest fever is a bad thing, rather than a welcome detox from something much more terrible.

Our ancestors, for thousands of years have developed immune systems that live in communion with all life. Through years of malnutrition and exposure to environmental poisons, this system has become weakened. Add to this vaccinations and other poisons and our species is facing extinction where the infertility rate, in our state (Utah), is now one in seven. This is getting worse.

Consider the words of Dr. Natasha Campbell-McBride, a practicing Neurologist and Neurosurgeon, and the world's foremost authority on the relationship of the developing gut and brain of a child and its immune system:

> *"Why does diarrhea reduce dramatically after a virus? I don't believe this theory that humanity has subscribed to for hundreds of years, which nature works on survival of the fittest. Nature works in cooperation. Every bug that comes to us our body has been invited. There is some job it needs to do for us. So every cold that we get, every virus, every flu that we get, is necessary. They come as cleansers, they come as purgers, they will come and remove something from your body, which if left in your body will cause something far more serious, far more terrible. So every viral infection is a blessing. Every cold is a blessing. It should not be fought and it should not be medicalized. So viruses do us a favor."* - GAPS CGP Conference, Indianapolis, Indiana, November 11th, 2014, www.gaps.me

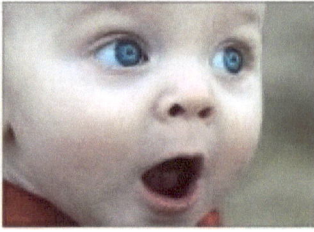

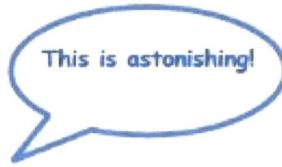

There's not a whole lot to say after Dr. McBride's comments. Bacteria and virus' "are our friends?!" Didn't you just take a deep breath of relief and release all that pent up fear the medical community has instilled in us?

When considering the community of life we live in, one can better appreciate the marvelousness of our immune response every time we come across an unfamiliar entity. Our immune system knows what to do. We do not need to force it into an unnatural reaction. This does not mean we cannot support the immune system through proper nutrition and supplementation that is designed to enhance the immune response.

In our clinic we have found the use of our 6-3-6 Immune Triad Protocol Podcast Episode #3 (http://traffic.libsyn.com/forbiddendoctor/03_FDPE03_ _The_Healing_Triad.mp3) to be amazingly effective boosting our immune strength. These three products, calcium lactate, whole food vitamin C, and an essential fatty acid found in whole food vitamin F, have been the staples of our clinic's approach to building immune strength for over a decade. More information about the

6-3-6 Immune Triad, can be found on our website, www.jackstockwell.com.

If you are like us, you are very grateful for many things in modern day medicine. Our problem is with the medical approach that criminalizes anything outside of "drugs for everything, drugs for anything." We would not want to see the elimination of any one drug or surgery that was necessary.

Our problem rests with the continued persecution and prosecution of those with proven methods of health restoration that do not fall within the arena of Big Pharma. For instance, you are not allowed to read our "Clinical Guide" because it does not have the sanction of the FDA. And the reason it will never have that is because, there are diseases listed and the nutrients that could help those conditions. *Gasp* you are not "allowed" to know this! This is the realm of the Forbidden Doctor, to bring these secrets into the open.

We are not trying to imply that your primary care physician has anything else in mind but your best interests, well-being and improved health. Historically, oriental doctors were only paid if they kept their patients well. If their patients got sick they weren't paid. So what were they motivated to do? Keep you well. Whereas western doctors only get paid when we get sick.

So what is the system set up to do? Keep you sick by only addressing the symptoms and not the cause of disease. There is no money in prevention in western medicine. Now, it's not the doctors per se, they are

good people, it's the way the system is set up, where the standard of care is established by the FDA and the pharmaceutical companies (who direct medical school curriculum), the AMA, and a whole army of government regulatory and bureaucratic agencies, that do not allow even a hint of foundational healing that goes to the source of the problem, rather than just the management of the symptoms. For instance, one might go to a cardiologist for high blood pressure only to receive a prescription for drugs to chemically force the pressure down, rather than going to the cause of the high blood pressure. We don't have healers coming out of medical schools anymore, instead we have chemical interventionists - "...where we are giving the patients poisons to correct the problems of starvation."
– Dr. Royal Lee. (www.seleneriverpress.com)

We leave you with an incredible bonus video of a speech by Robert F. Kennedy Jr., before a crowd of angry, sorrowful, heartbroken and demanding mothers, whose children have been seriously injured by vaccines.

Robert F. Kennedy exposing the truth

Present Robert F Kennedy Jr Shocking Vaccine Cover Up Part 1

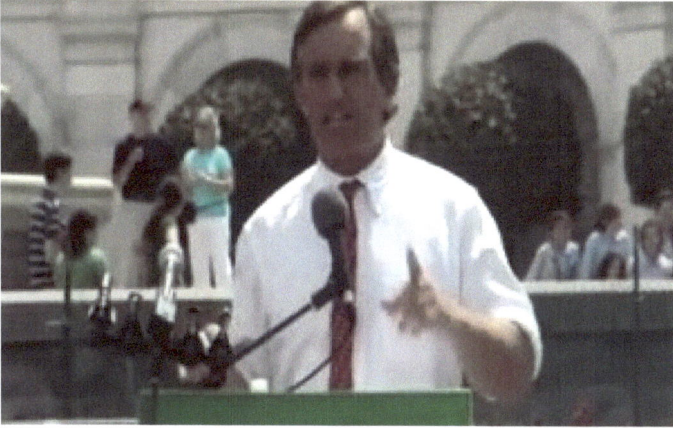

Type in this URL in your web browser to view the video on YouTube:

https://www.youtube.com/watch?v=UQG5Q4GWw2o

Present Robert F Kennedy Jr Shocking Vaccine Cover Up Part 2

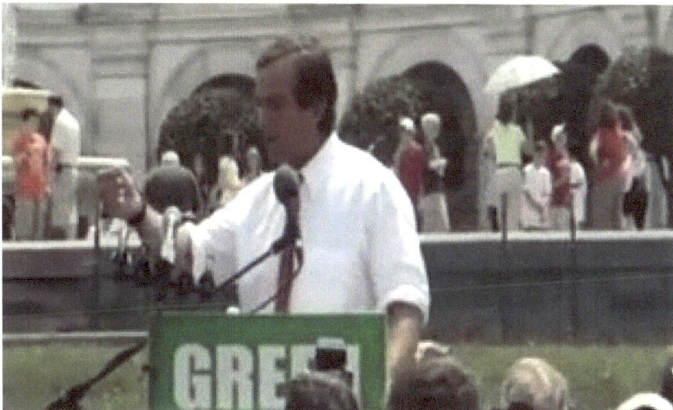

Type in this URL in your web browser to view the video on YouTube:

https://www.youtube.com/watch?v=DjPox5xBOLI

If you really want to have some fun, type in the URL address below the magazine cover.

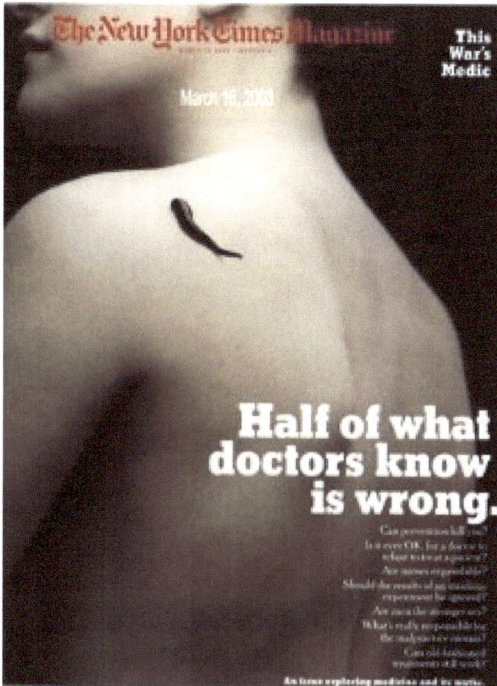

"....half of what we teach you
here is wrong -- unfortunately,
we don't know which half."

Browser URL Link:
http://www.nytimes.com/2003/03/16/magazine/16INT
RO.html

ABOUT THE AUTHORS

Dr. Jack is an Upper Cervical NUCCA Board Certified Chiropractor (nucca.org), one of only 27 on the planet! His practice and successes are the result of his painless, extremely effective, and lasting technique, the help of an amazing team behind him, and through his relentless research to learn all he can to make sure patients are receiving the absolute best.

Mary, along with her husband Jack, started the BioScan department in 2004. It evolved into a Personal Health Profiling & Nutritional Consulting department, giving people personalized nutritional help. After helping thousands of patients, from Fibromyalgia to Crohn's disease, she has reached a level of results that few have achieved.

Both Jack and Mary are GAPS Certified Practitioners (gaps.me). Together, they have over 33 years "talking health" on the radio. And are the creators of the "FORBIDDEN DOCTOR PODCAST." (http://www.forbiddendoctor.com) Mary and Jack currently live in Draper, Utah.

To learn more about them and their clinic, visit their websites: http://www.jackstockwell.com/ and http://www.forbiddendoctor.com/.

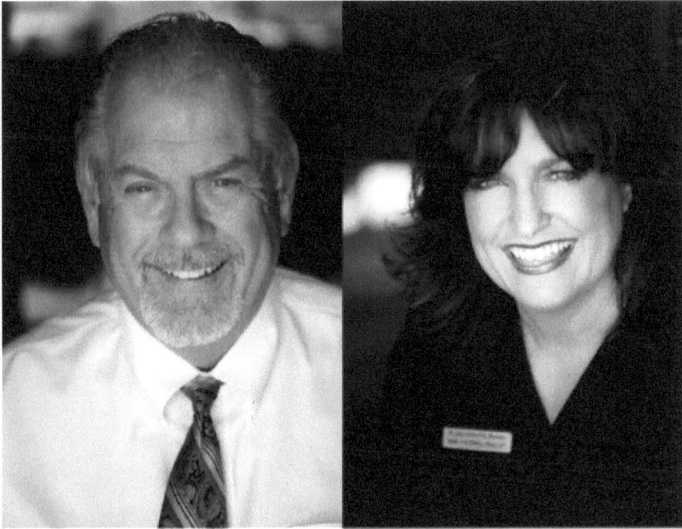

We hope you learned something from what we have just shared. We have been fortunate enough to be able to put this e-book together and have put ourselves out there is hopes that the truth will be shed some light.

We would be honored if you reviewed this book on Amazon (http://amzn.to/1U5bfG3). Thank you.

www.ingramcontent.com/pod-product-compliance
Lightning Source LLC
Chambersburg PA
CBHW041720200326
41521CB00001B/137